Bad burning diarrhea or did you eat spicy foods that burn

Solution: Cool the area by hitting it with cool water from your shower. You can use your hand or a washcloth to guide the cool water on the anal area. If you do not have a shower, you can run cool water from your bathtub and use a washcloth on the area.

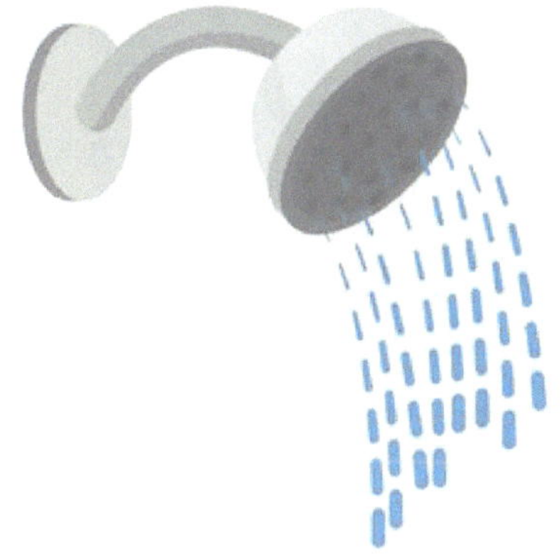

Certain headaches

Solution: Stop eating and drinking foods with nitrates in them. Foods and drinks with nitrates such as apple juice and hot dogs can cause headaches.

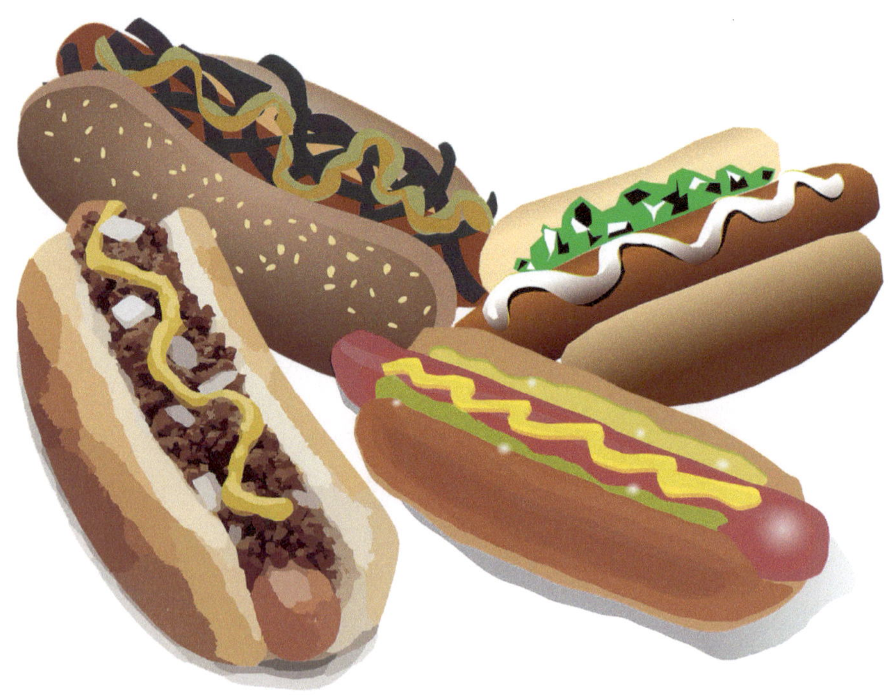

Bad gas or an upset stomach

Solution: Drink a lemon-lime soda.

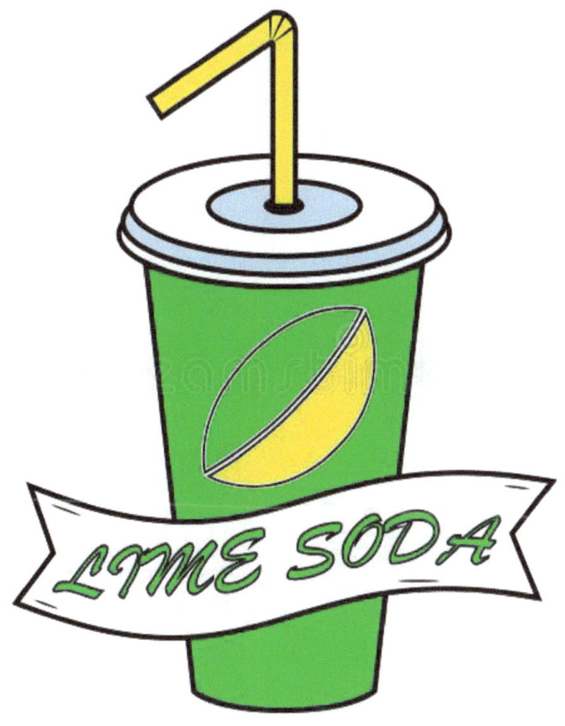

Tooth and or/ cavity pain

Solution: Put all-natural unsweetened applesauce on the tooth or in the broken tooth to stop the pain. You should be pain-free while the applesauce is in the pain area. Make sure to buy a good amount of applesauce because it will dissolve quickly. My advice to you is to have a bag or a bucket near you to spit out the applesauce if you do not want to eat it.

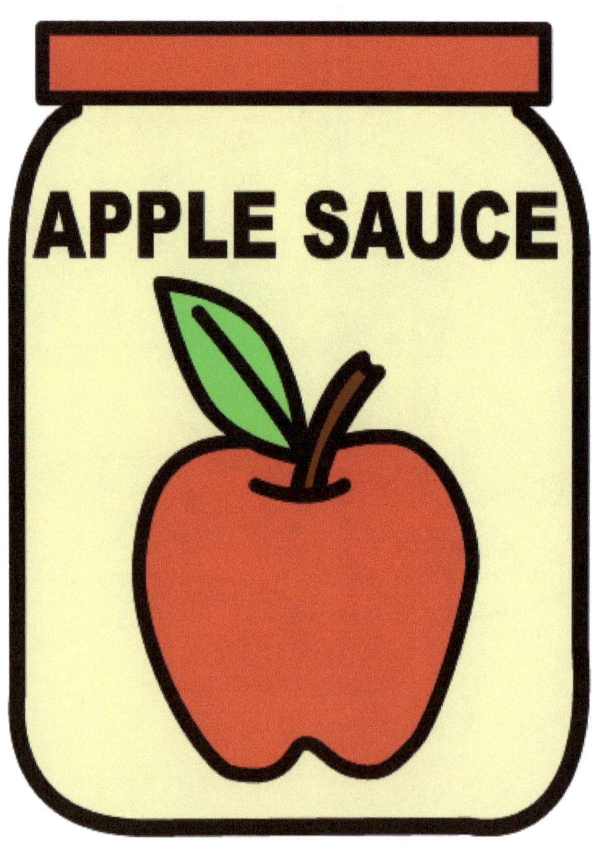

Foot and/ or ankle pain

Solution: Wear thick-bottom sandals/ house shoes. The thick cushioned shoe brand sandals work the best.

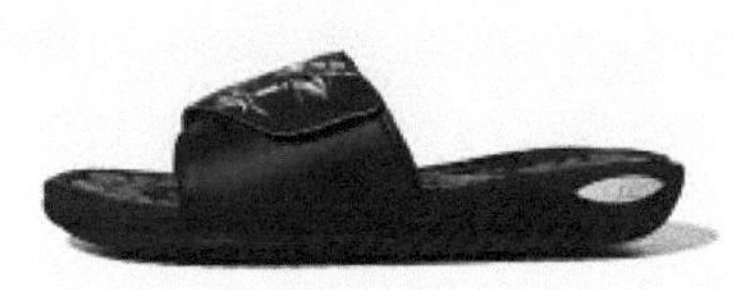

Open certain locked doors when locked out

Solution: Slide a credit card, driver's license, or photo identification card between the locks and open the door. To be more clear, swipe the card between the lock that is keeping the door closed and the lock that is installed on the wall or the side panel on the wall/ door opening.

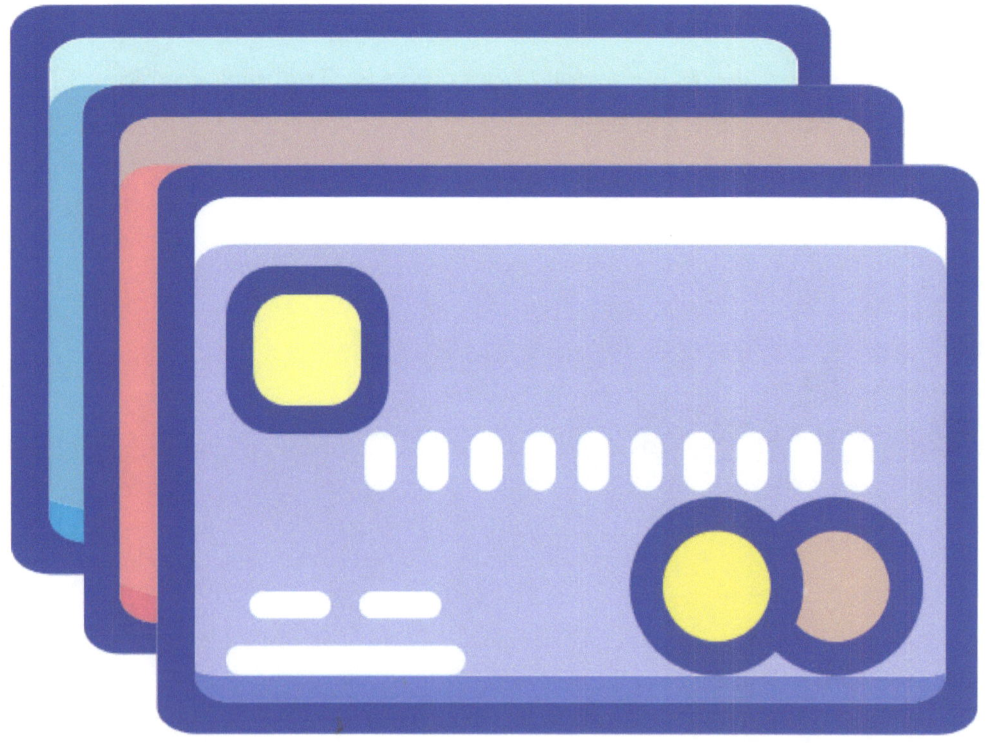

Get rid of lower back pain

Solution: Put your leg opposite of the side with the back pain on the bathtub or on a sturdy chair, squat down with the opposite arm side, put the arm between your legs and hold the pose for 15-20 seconds. You should be imitating a Quarterback hiking a football but holding the pose.

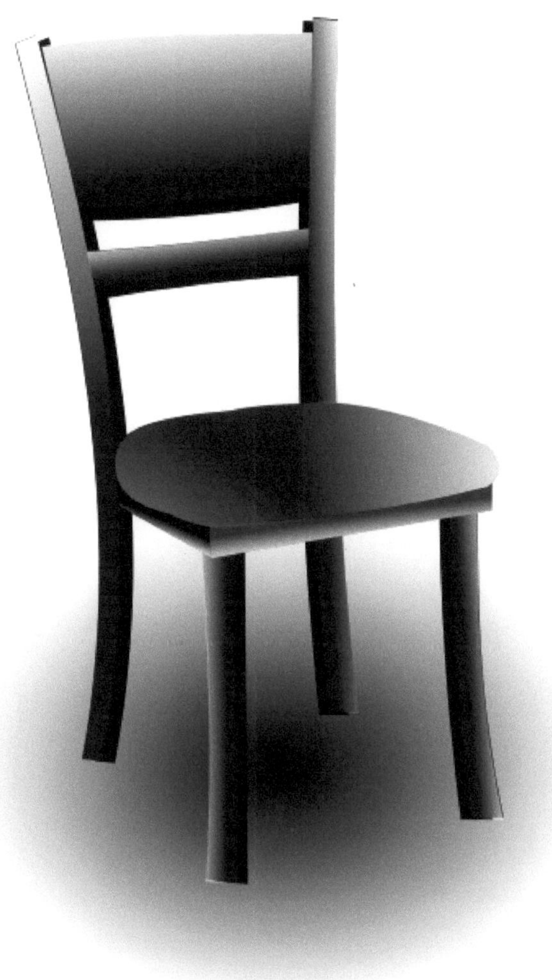

Leg and thigh cramps

Solution: Drink a sports drink. If you regularly get cramps, try drinking one sports drink a day plus plenty of water. Eating bananas is also a good option.

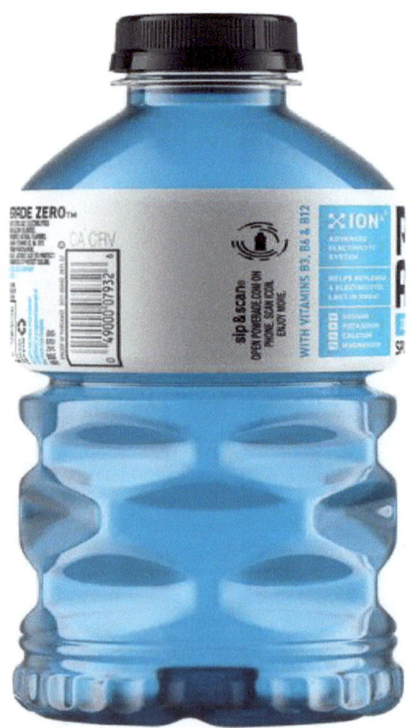

Remove a tight sticky bandage

Solution: Slowly pull the bandage off while water from your sink or shower hits the area between your skin and the bandage. The water will help the bandage peel off. For difficult bandages where bleeding may occur, use saline on the bandage to loosen it up for removal.

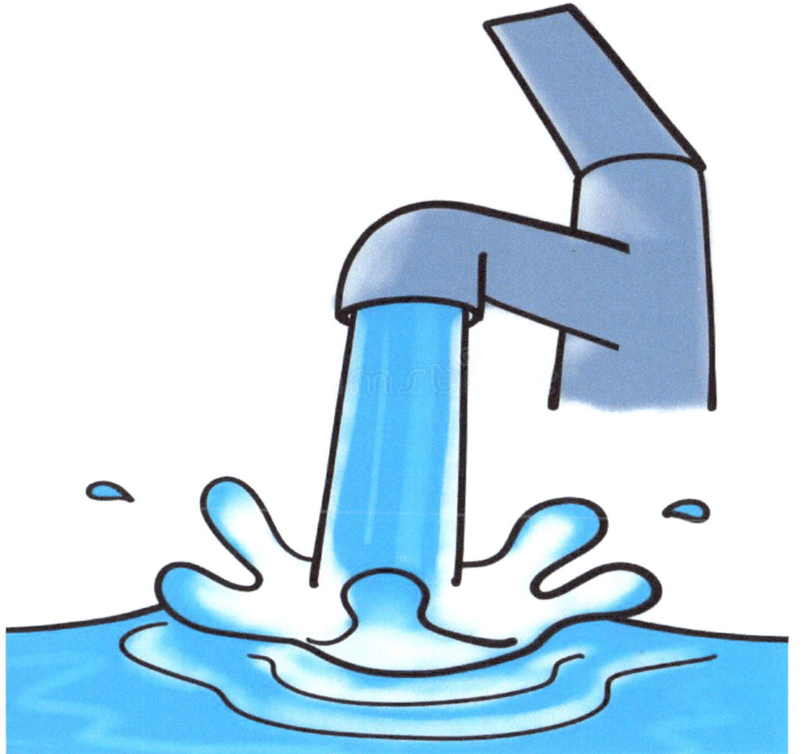

Soothe burning toes

Solution: Put your burning toes on a metal chair. The metal will cool down the burning sensation. Keep your toes on the chair as long as needed. Repeat when the burning returns.

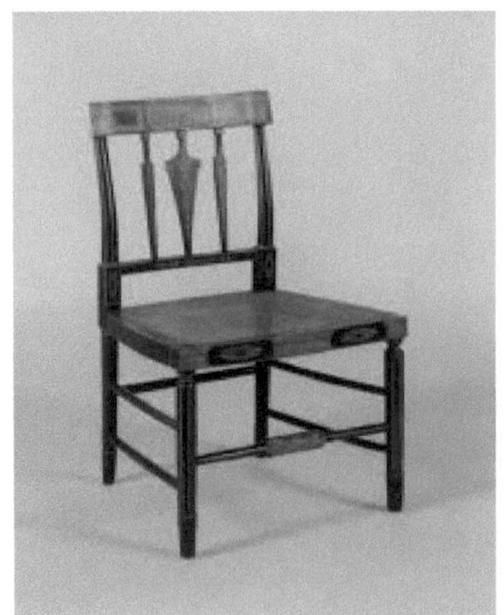

Treat painful swollen gums

Solution: A lemon can get the swelling down by placing it on the swollen area. Take the lemon off the area when you see a little blood. The swelling should continue going down and draining through the bleeding area. **Note: Please consult with a dentist or medical professional first.**

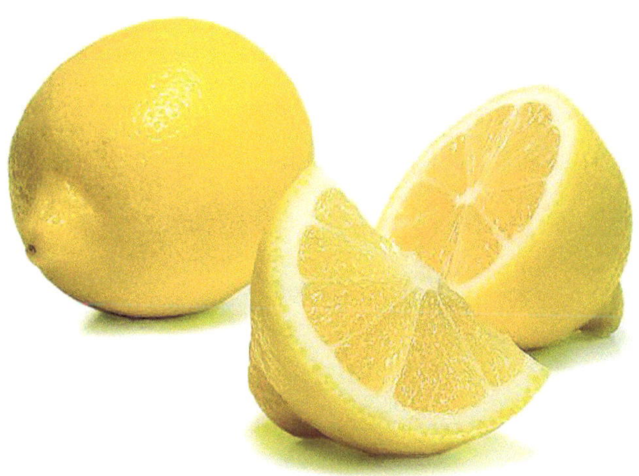

Relieve stomach acid

Solution: Eat kiwis.

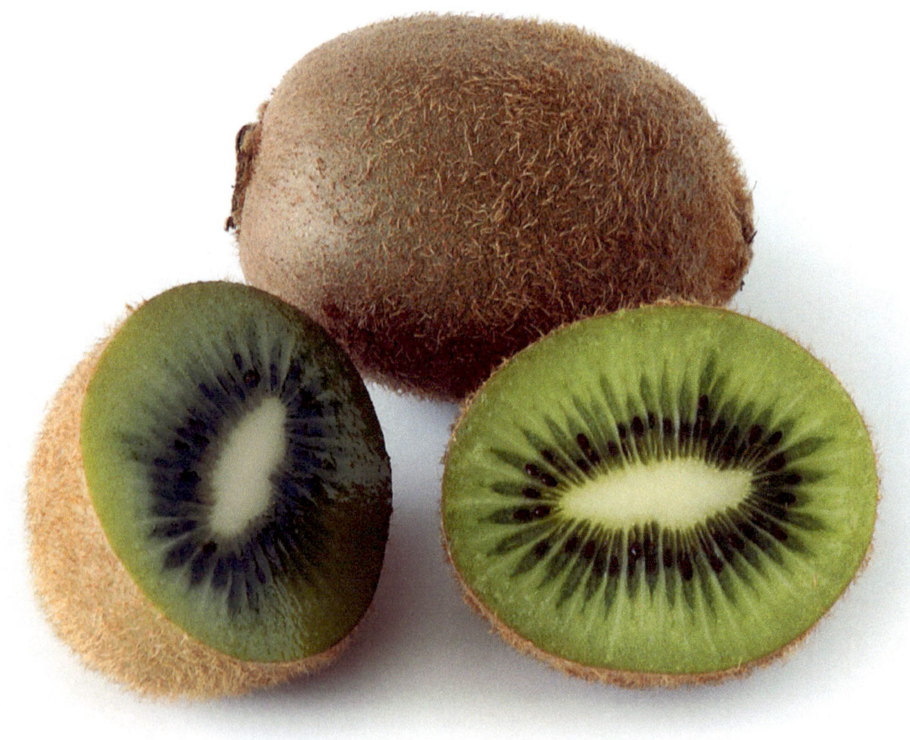

Reduce sinus congestion

Solution: Eat blueberries. If blueberries do not work try eating some spicy food or onions. In some cases, wearing a mask or an N95 respirator could help if the congestion is caused by air quality.

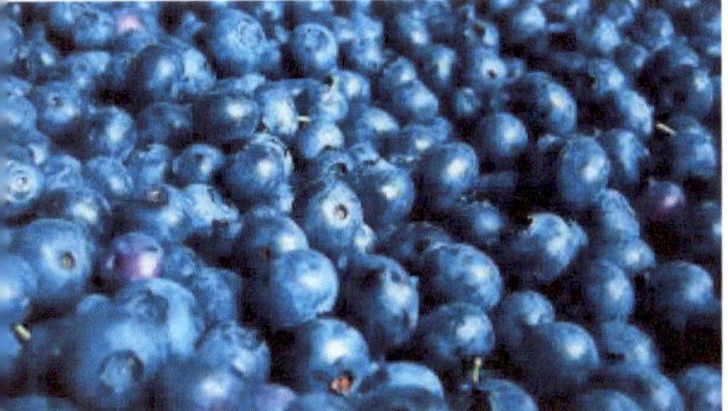

Make a magnifying glass

Solution: Hold your prescription or store-bought glasses six inches away from your face and look through the lens at the writing or item you want to see.

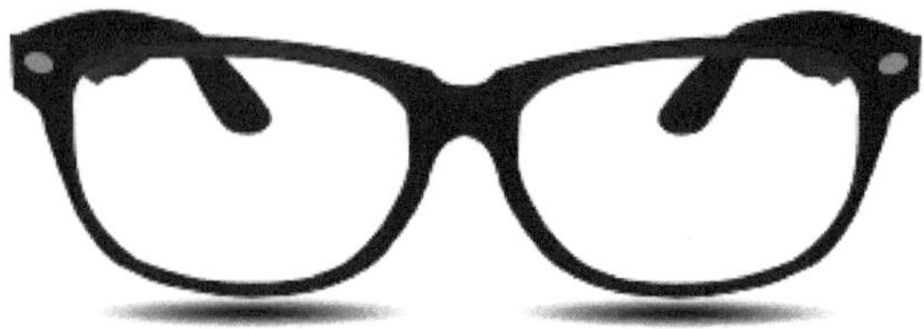

Lower your blood pressure

Solution: Eat natural diuretic foods such as watermelon and blueberries to help release sodium from your body. Drinking grape juice and eating some chocolate could also help.

Please contact your doctor or a medical professional on the steps you should take to manage your blood pressure. The advice given is not to replace medical advice or to encourage skipping or not taking prescribed medications.

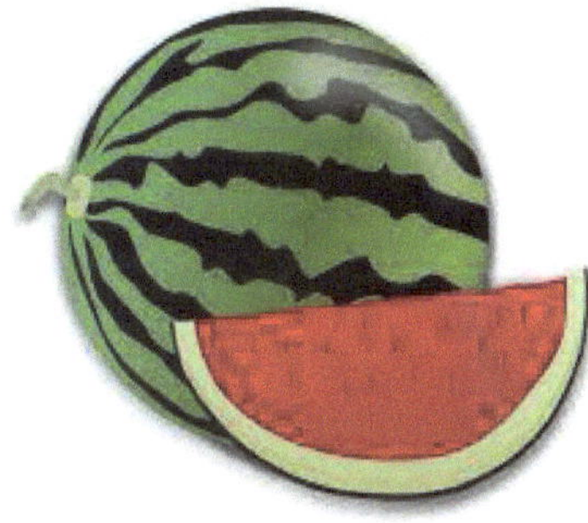

Stop bad bleeding until the paramedic arrives

Solution: The first thing to do is use a clean cloth and apply pressure to the wound until the paramedic arrives. If someone is there to assist you, put a gauze over the wound after the bleeding stops and wrap it with microfoam tape. An Israeli bandage could also be used to stop the bleeding. If you can't do either, use a clean washcloth and apply pressure to the wound until the paramedics arrive.

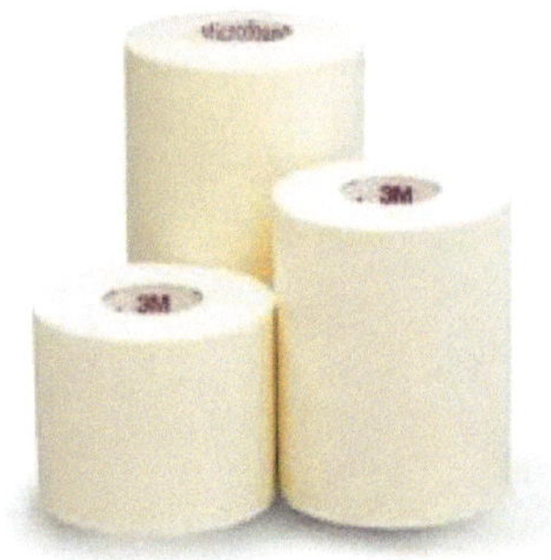

Get free cell phone service

Solution: You can apply for the Government's Lifeline free phone program for low-income people, receiving SNAP, food stamps, Medicaid, or other programs.

If neither of the above applies to you: You can download a free Wifi phone service app and use Wifi phone service whenever you are at a location with free Wifi. Some of the Wifi phone apps offer cheap full cell phone service as well.

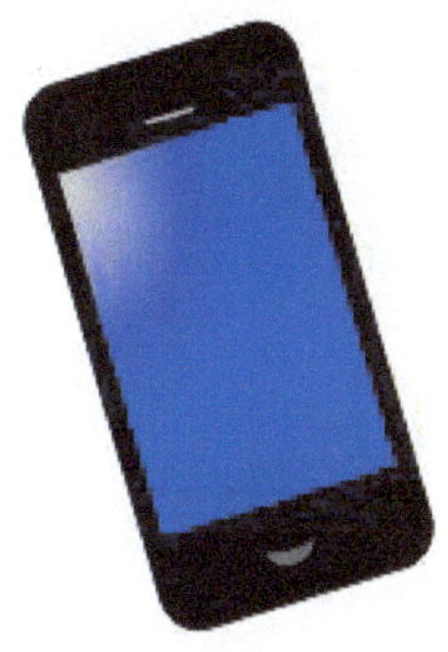

Get your leftover food to keep its flavor

Solution: Freeze your leftovers in a storage or freezer bag. When you are ready to eat the leftovers, microwave, or use your oven or stovetop to warm up the food.

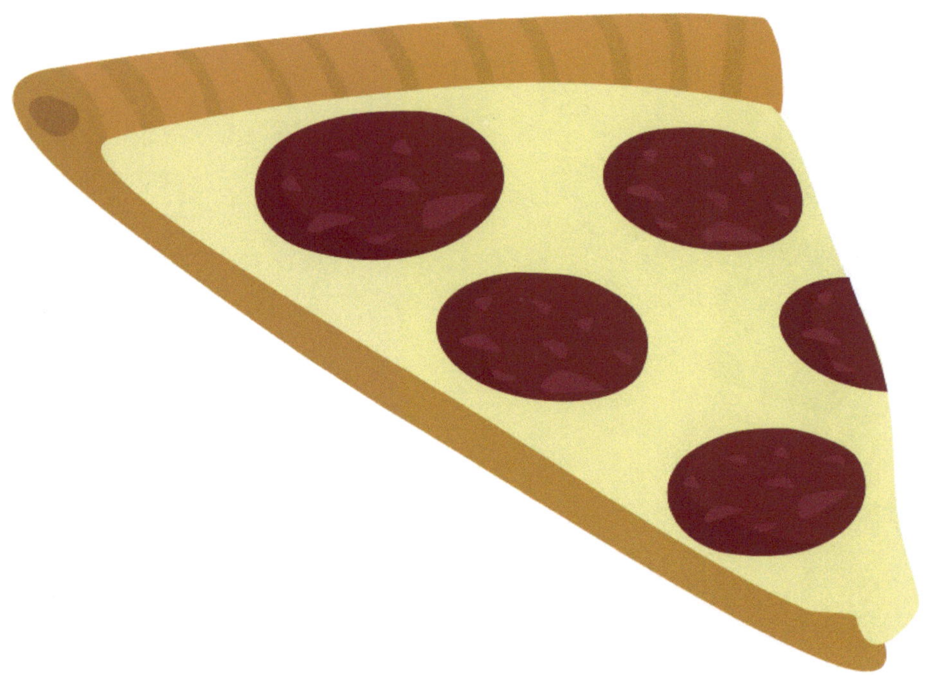

Remove a sticky candy wrapper

Solution: Put the candy or the bag of candy in the refrigerator for 20-30 minutes or in the freezer for 15 minutes.

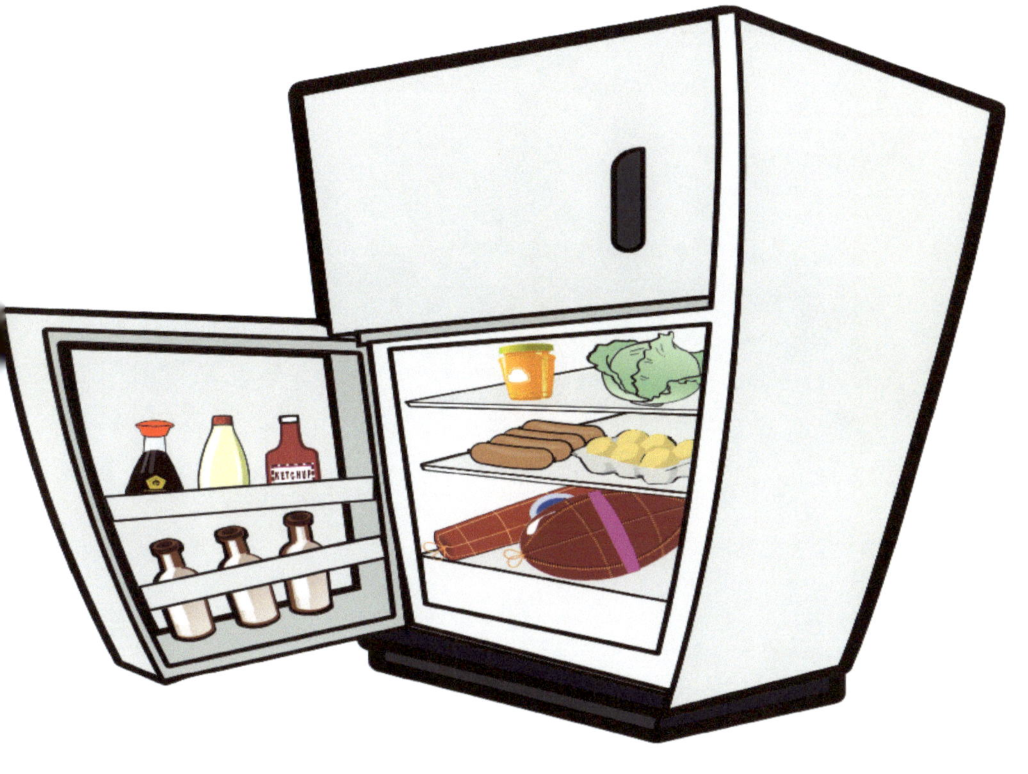

Get rid of the pain after cutting fingernails too short

Solution: Put a bandage over the fingernails that are in pain and let the bandage hang over the fingernail tip. If you are out of bandages, use tape. Using masking tape would be preferred.

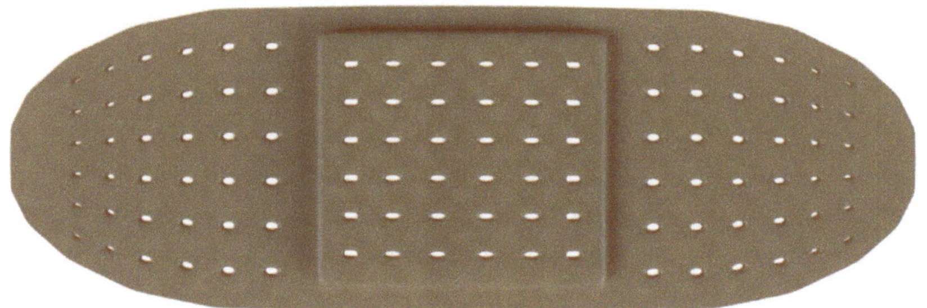

Relieve a sore throat

Solution: Suck on some hard candy such as butterscotch or peppermint candy.

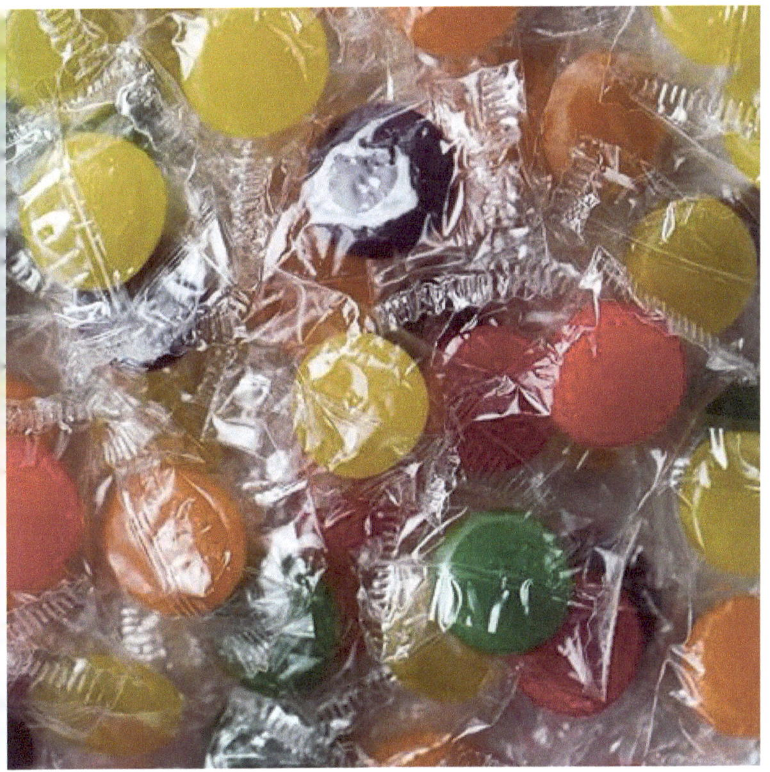

Get canceled Amazon Prime membership renewal to work right away after a payment

Solution: Buy an Amazon e-gift card from the website and load the amount of your Amazon Prime membership on it. Once received, use the gift card to pay for your Prime membership. You will be able to use the membership benefits right away instead of waiting for a credit card payment to process.

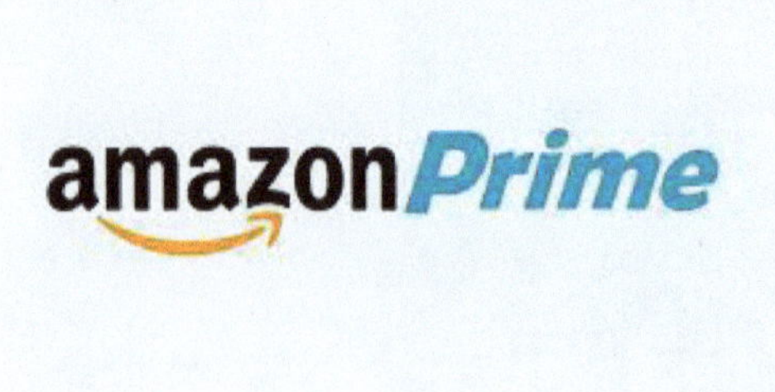

Thank you for your purchase. You can contact the author Tron Griffin at sol15g@yahoo.com . Please try his other books on Amazon and places where books are sold.

Tron's books include:

Danny and his Brown friend

The fight for Kisington

Surviving the South Side of Chicago

The House of Murders

Trust me, if you can

Flip to the next pages for bonus remedies.

Stop MSG, fried food, and certain chocolate from giving you palpitations/ high heart rate

Solution: Refrigerate the food for at least 30 minutes before consuming it.

Please consult with a doctor before trying this remedy.

Stop your heart from skipping a beat

Solution: Try a few pieces of chocolate.

Please consult with a doctor before trying this remedy.

9 798327 159631